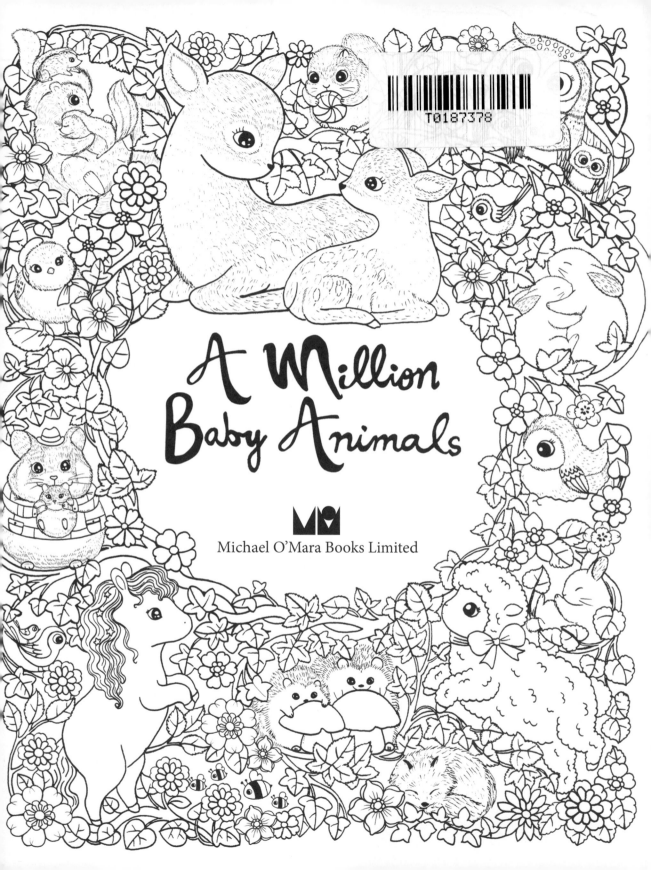

A Million Baby Animals

Michael O'Mara Books Limited

First published in Great Britain in 2024 by Michael O'Mara Books Limited,
9 Lion Yard, Tremadoc Road, London SW4 7NQ

W www.mombooks.com

f Michael O'Mara Books

y @OMaraBooks

O @omarabooks

A CIP catalogue record for this book is available from the British Library.

ISBN: 978-1-78929-524-5

3 5 7 9 10 8 6 4 2

This book was printed in China.

MIX
Paper | Supporting
responsible forestry
FSC® C010256
FSC
www.fsc.org

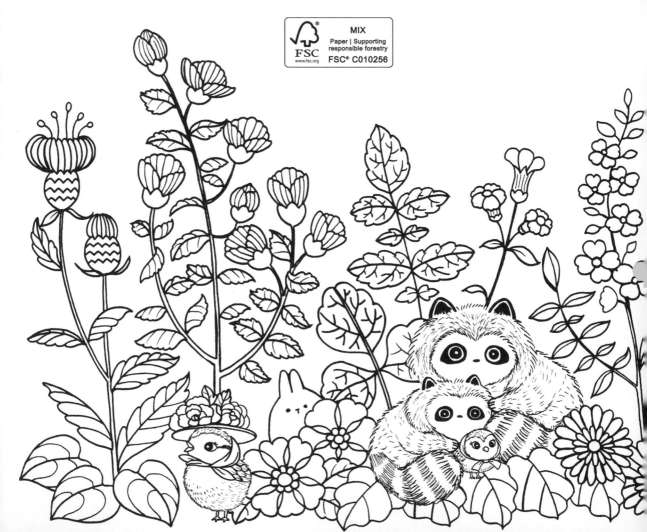

Illustrated by

Lulu Mayo

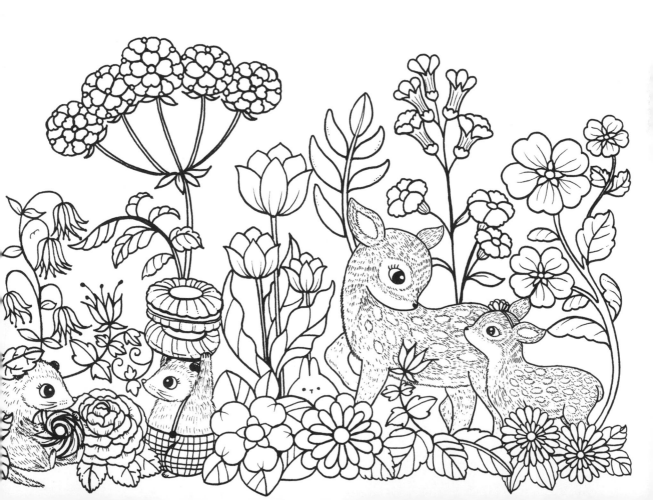

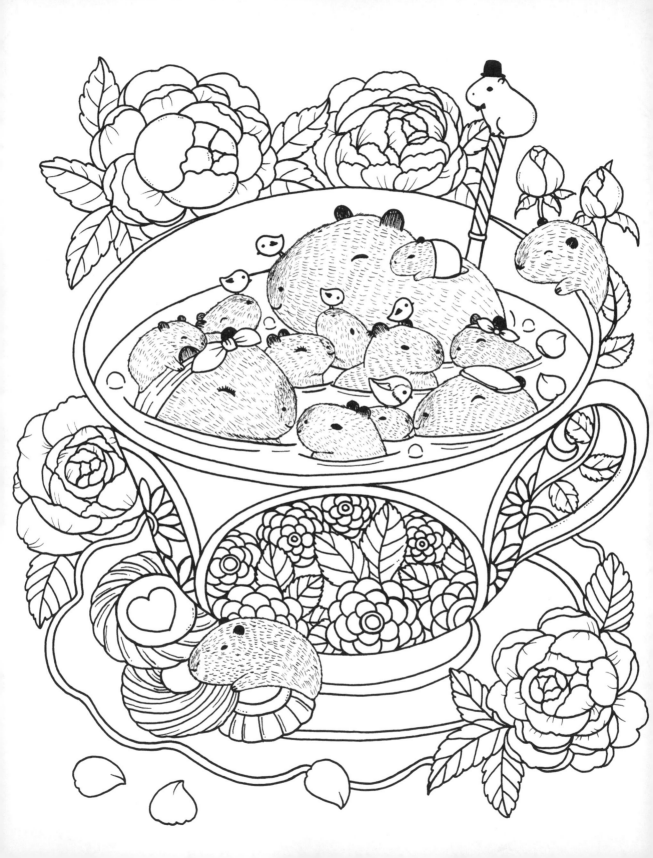

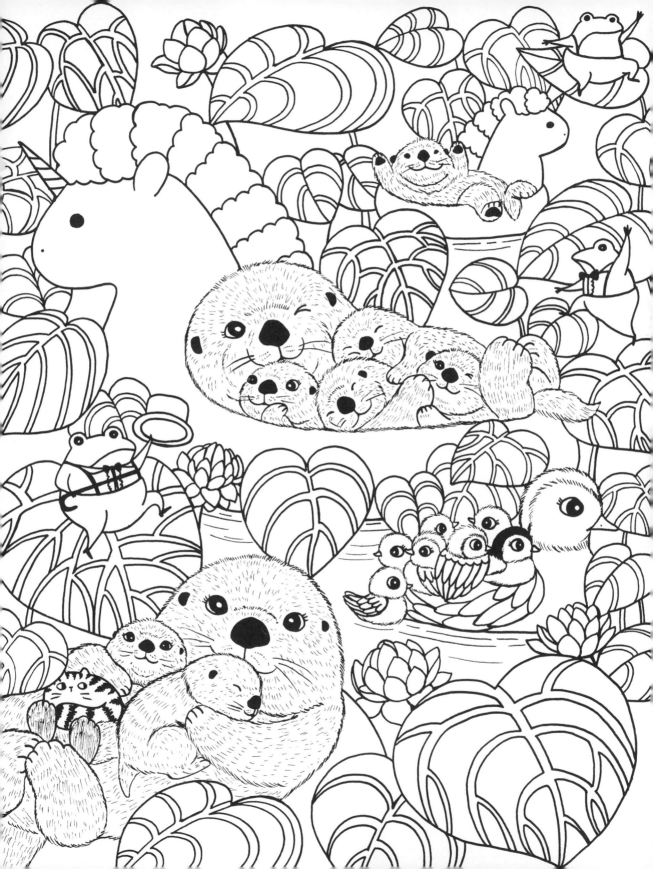

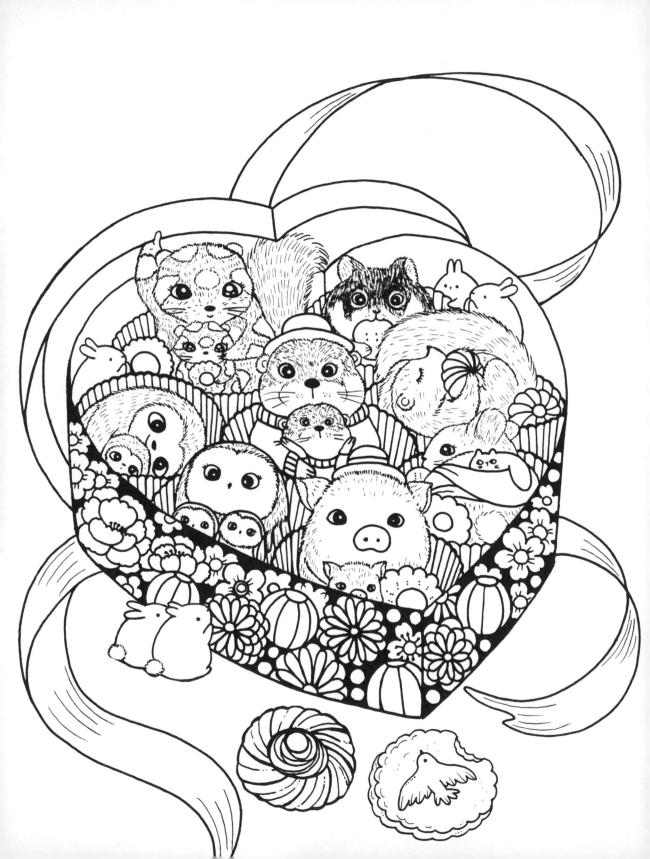

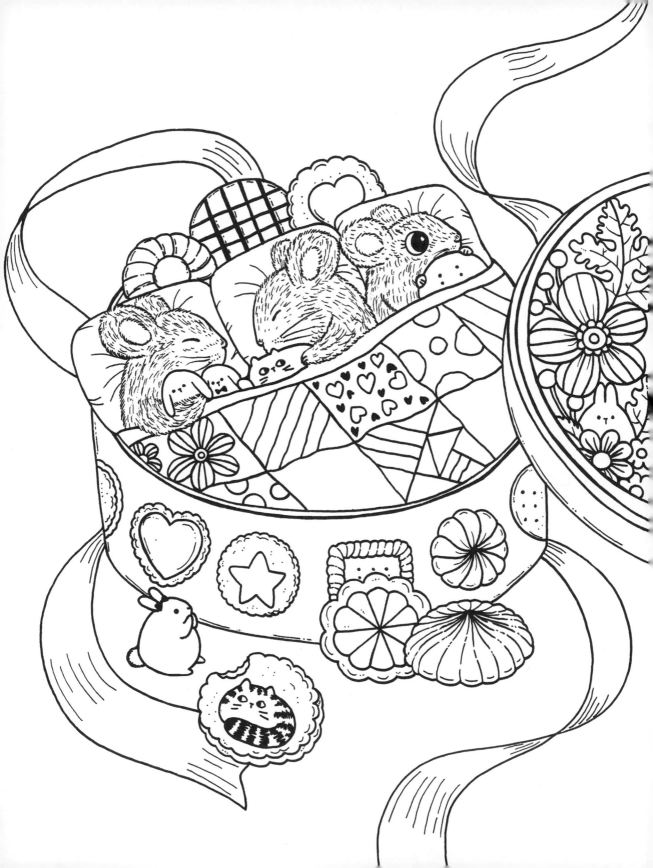

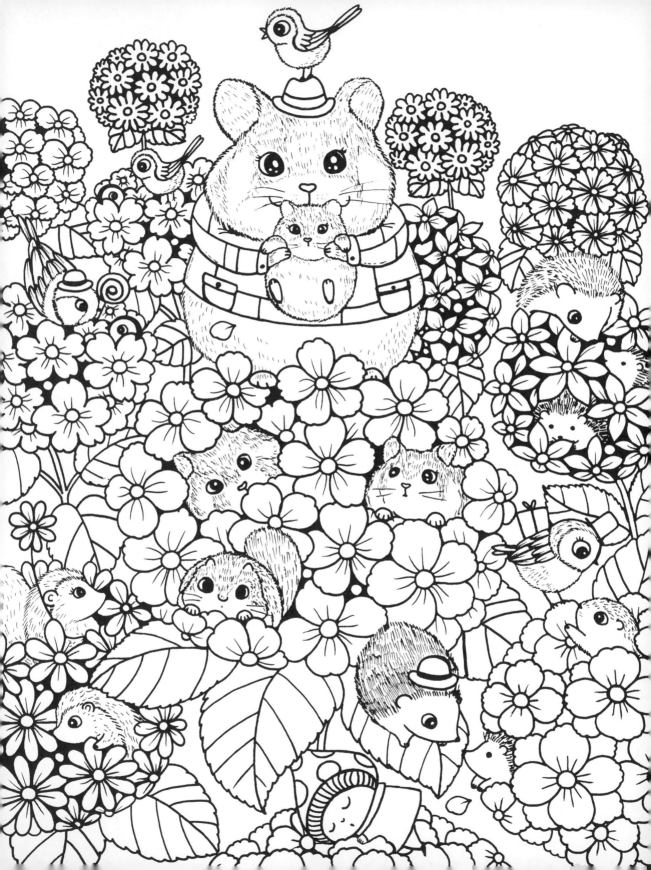

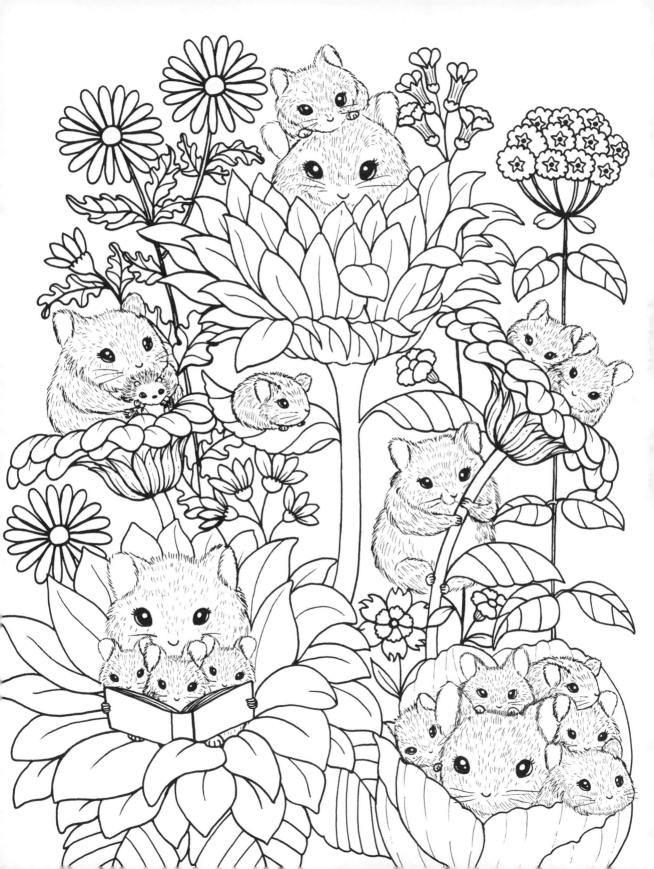

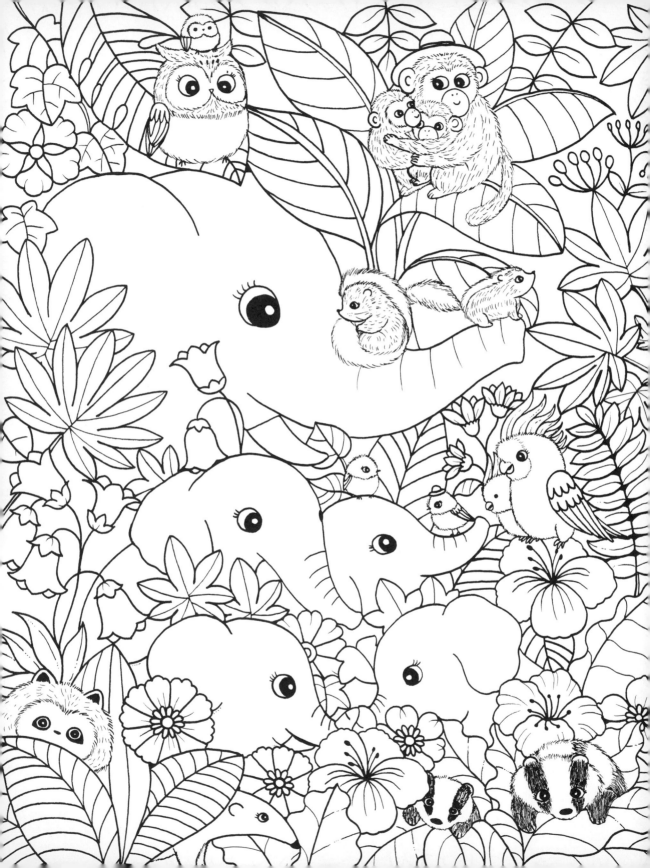

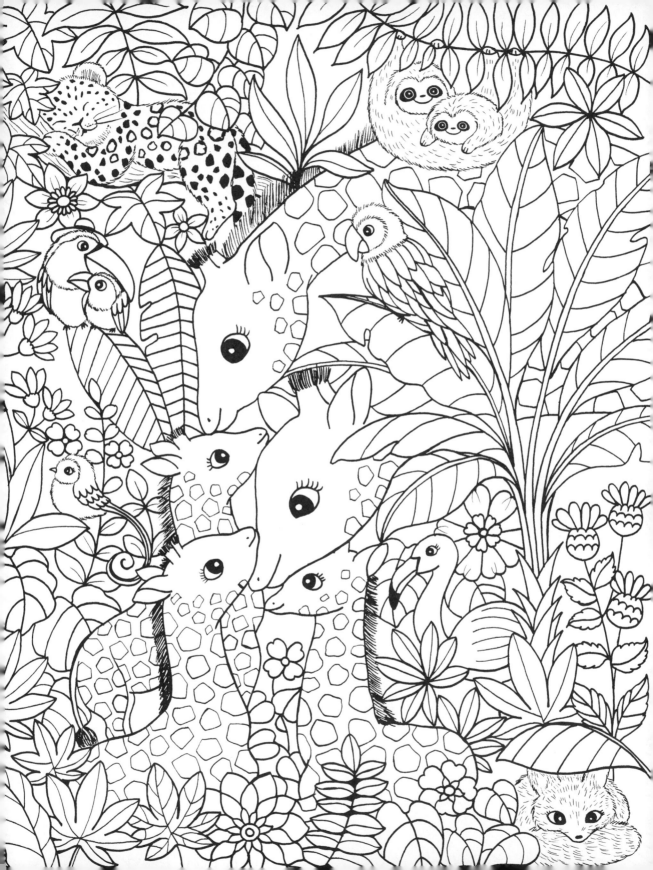

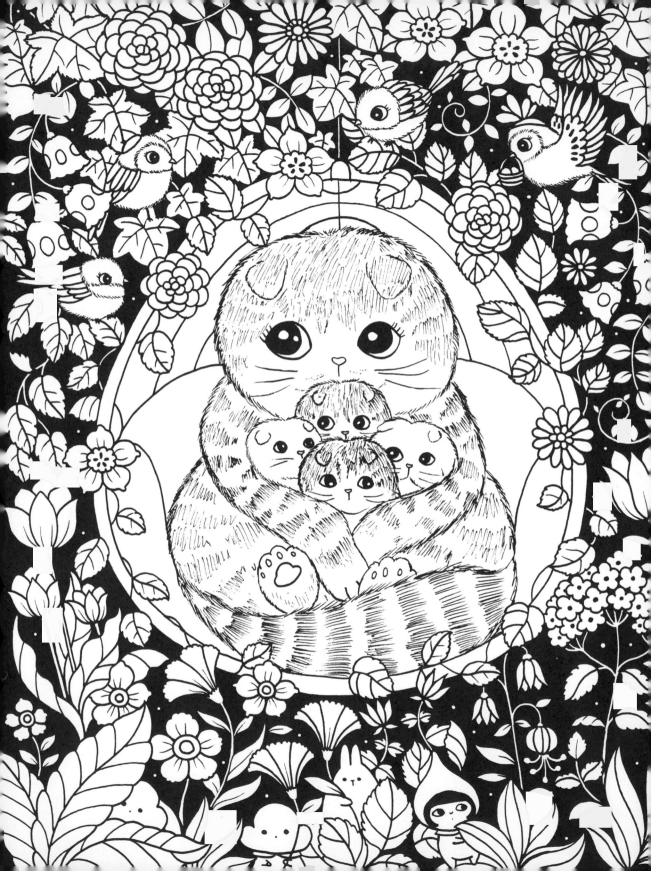

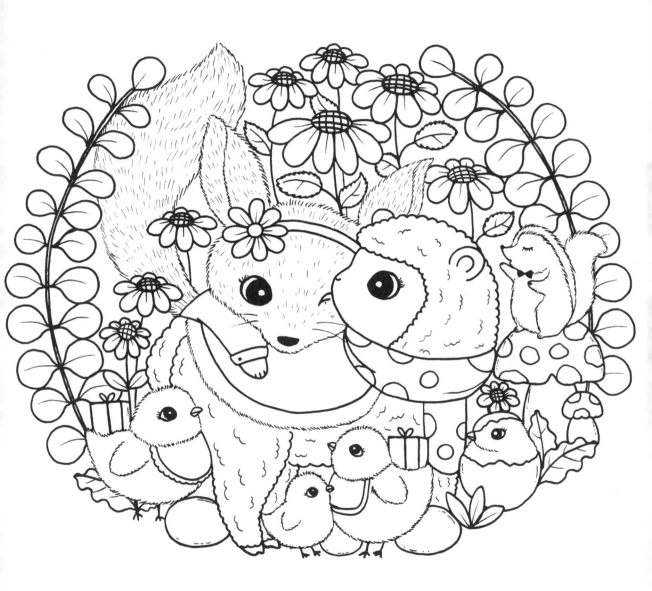

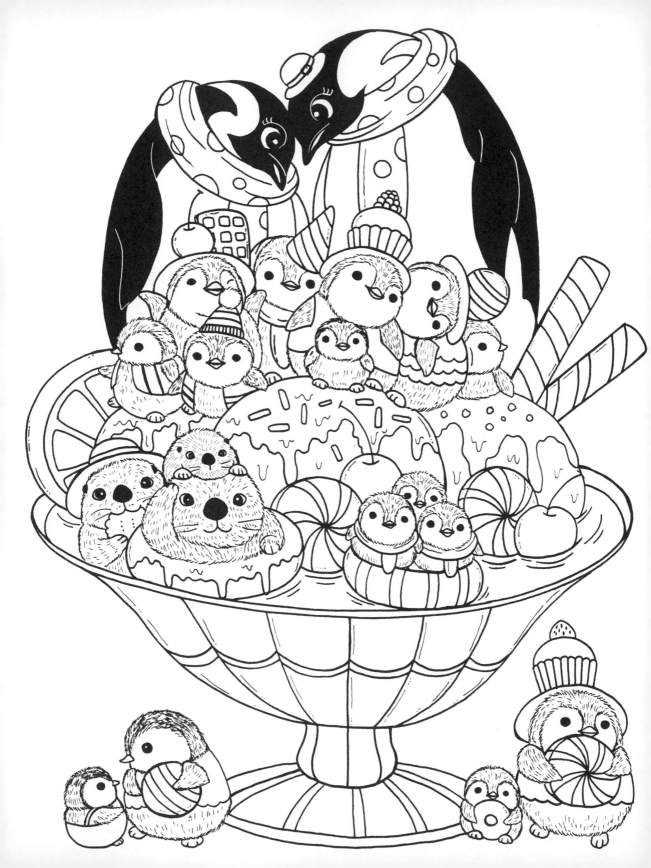

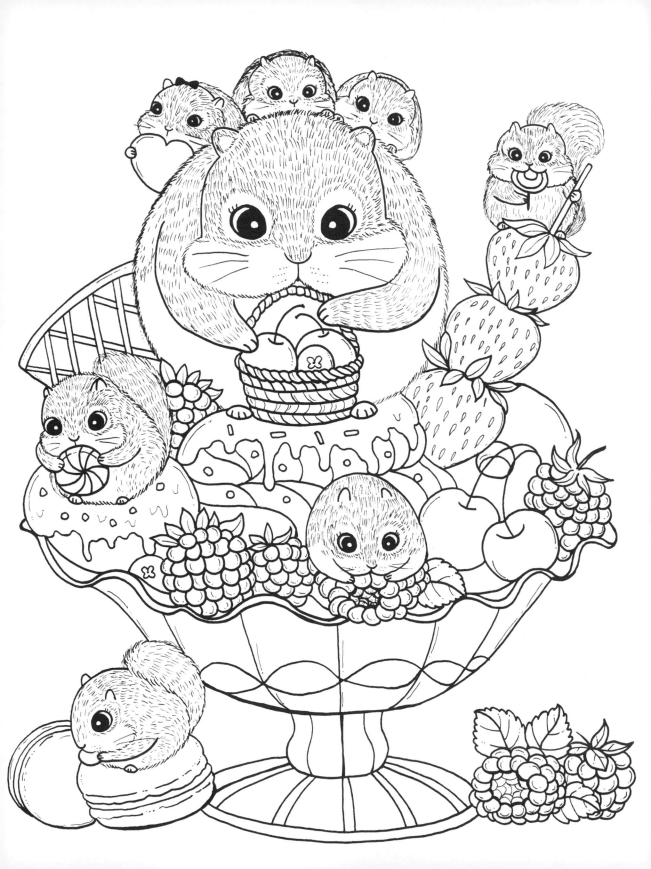

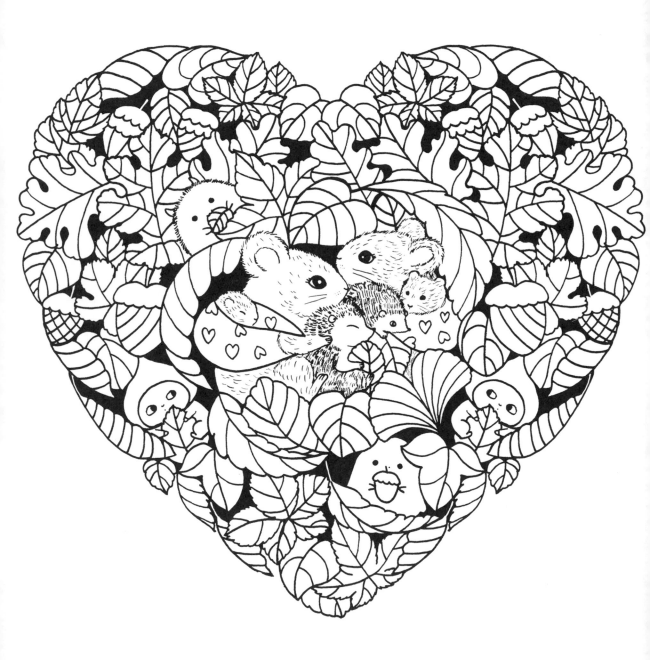

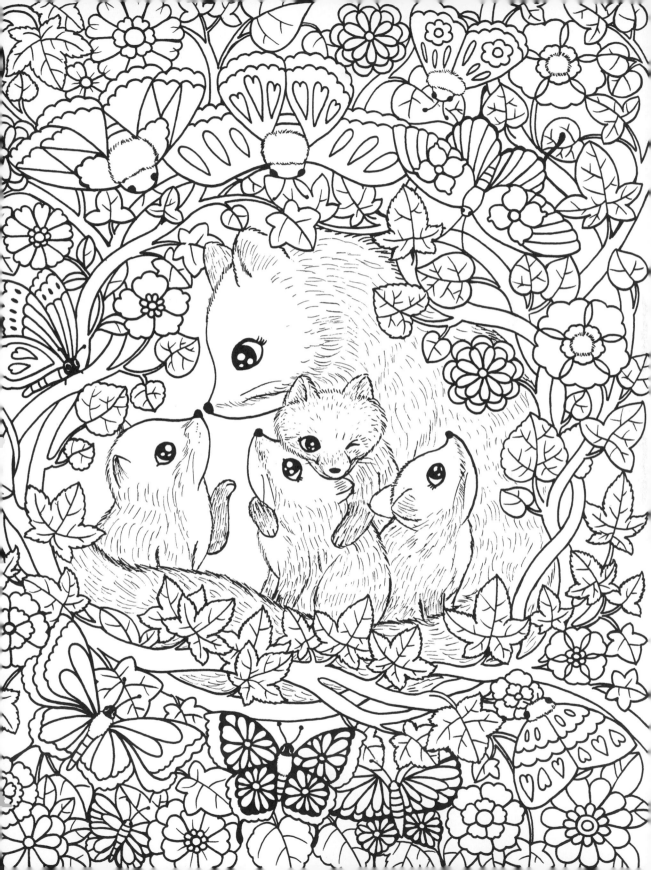

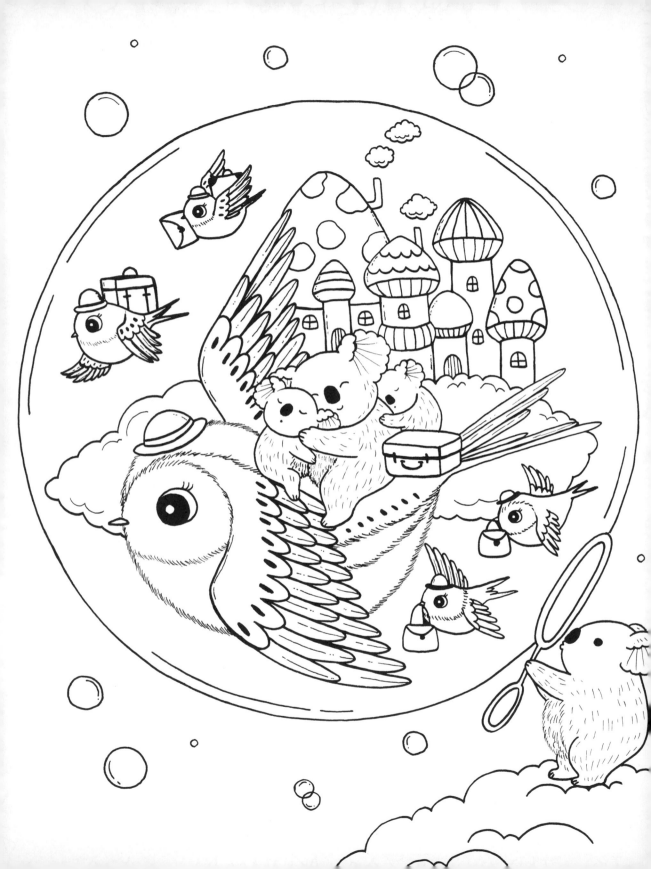

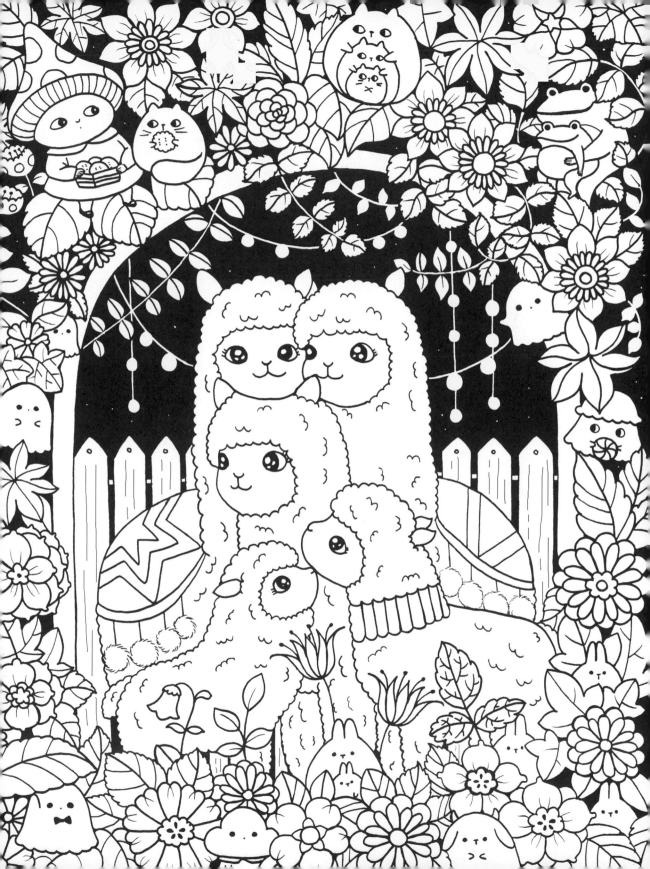

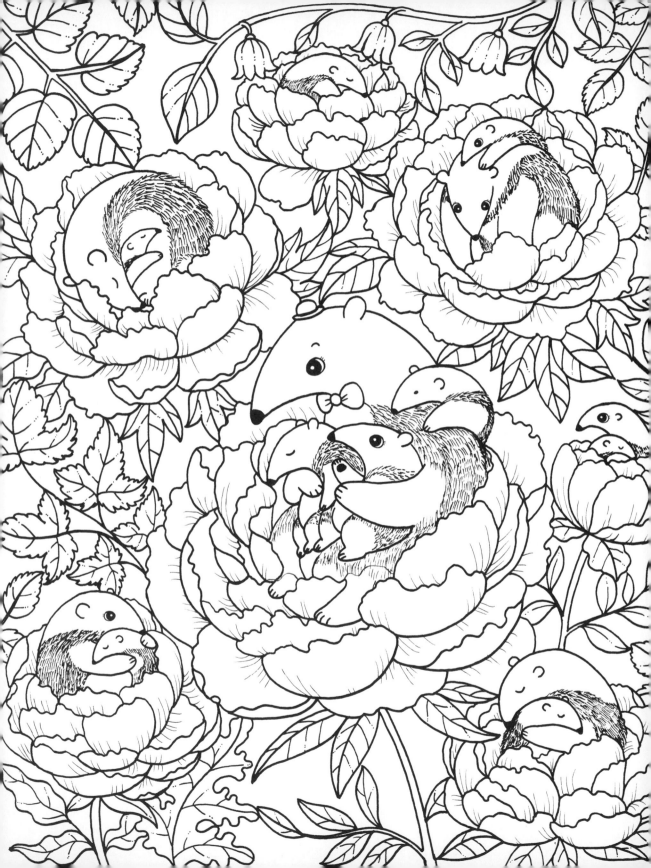

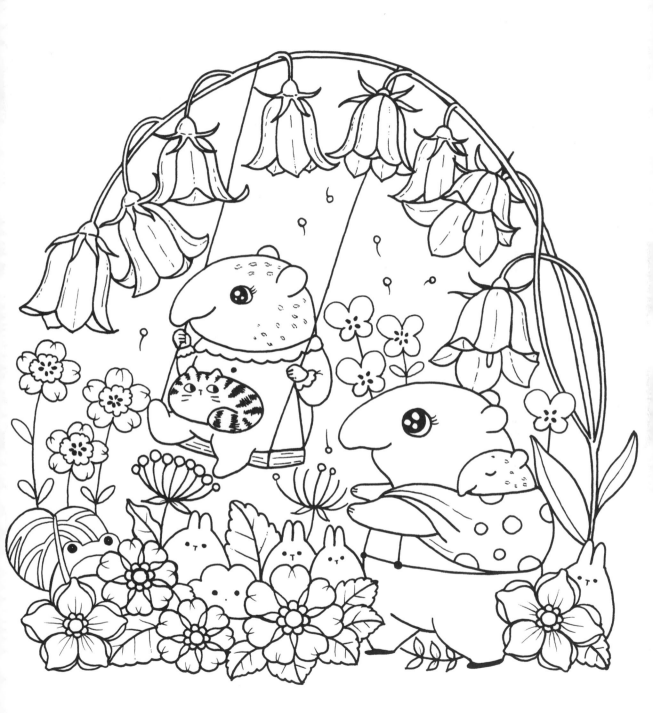

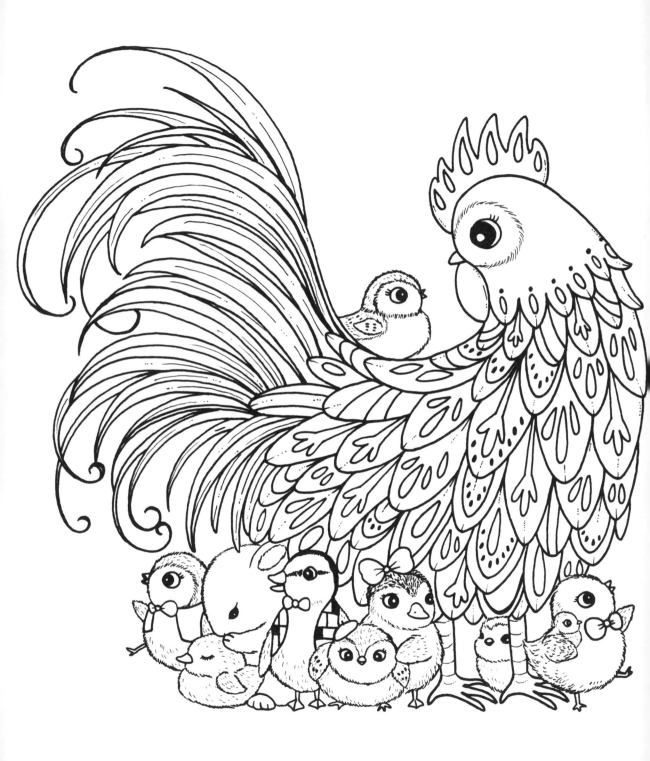

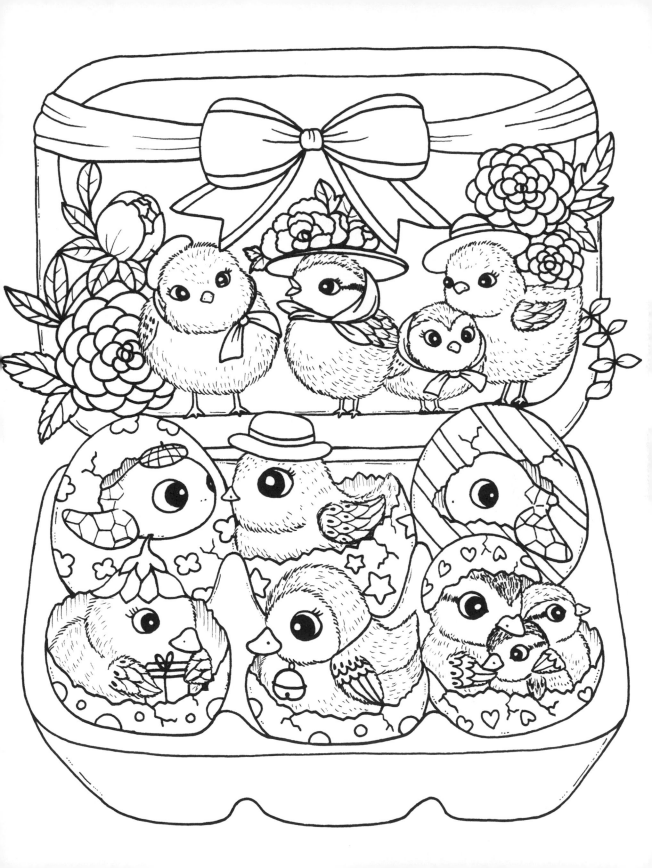

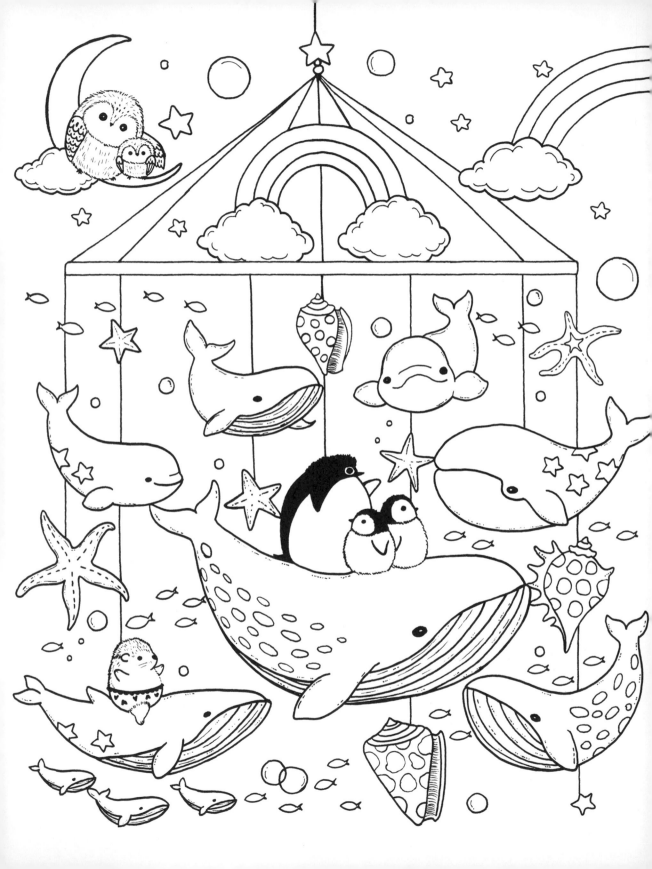

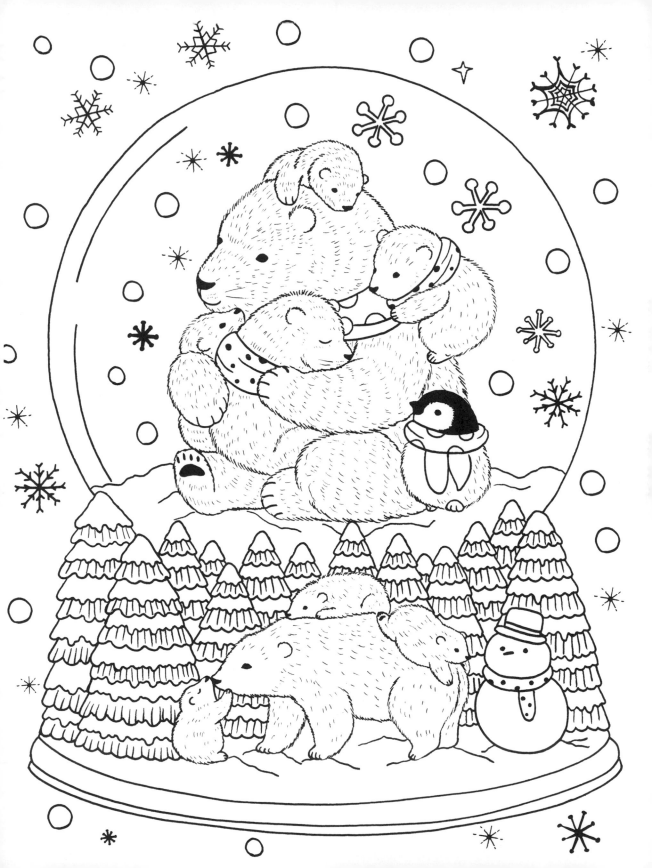

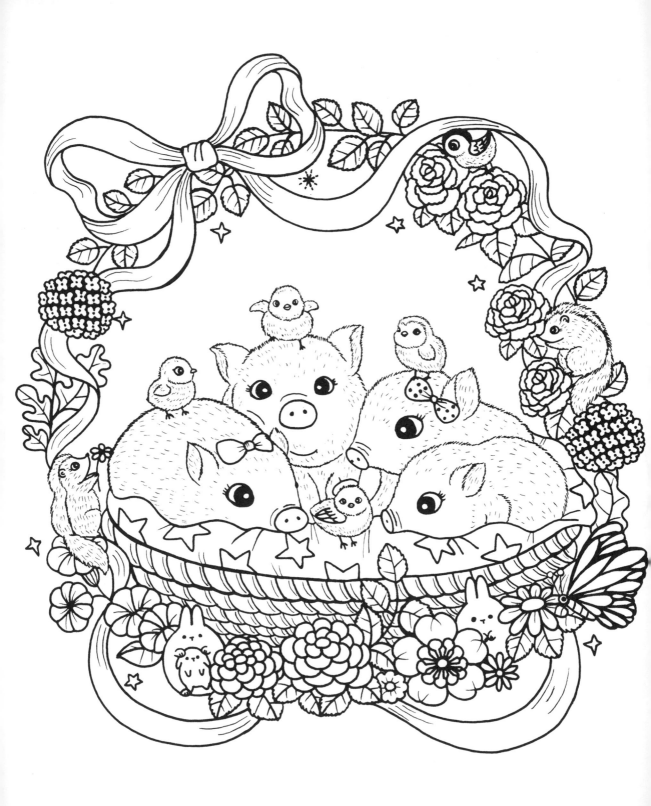

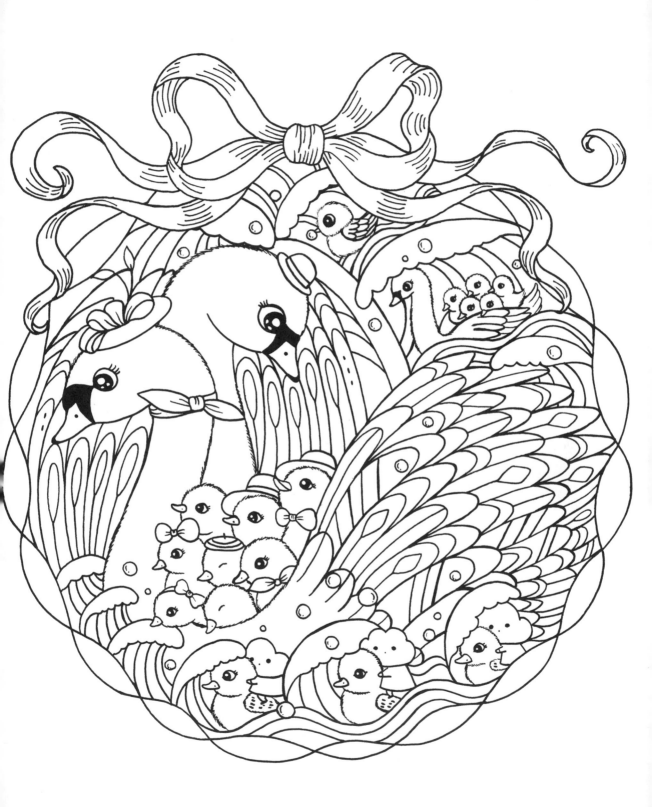

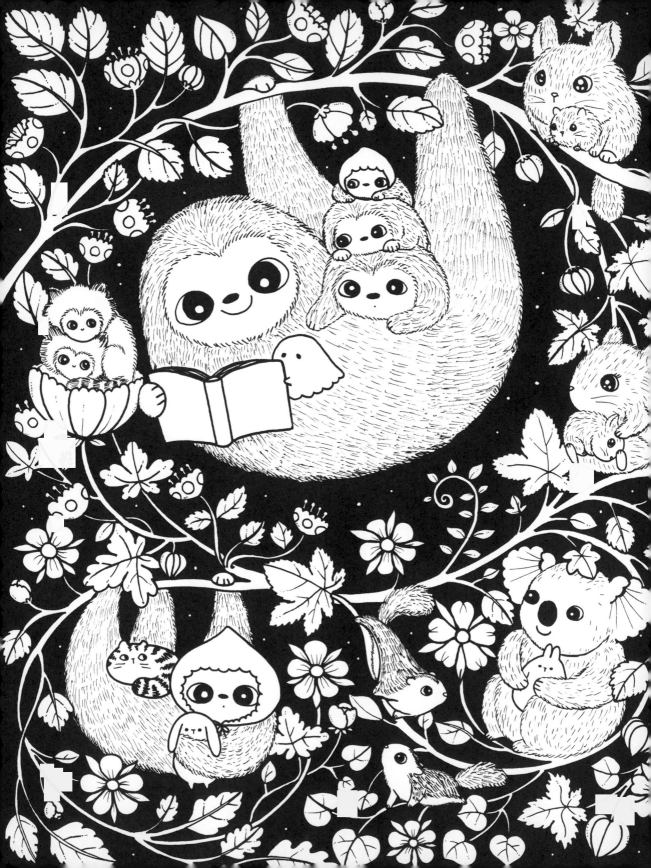

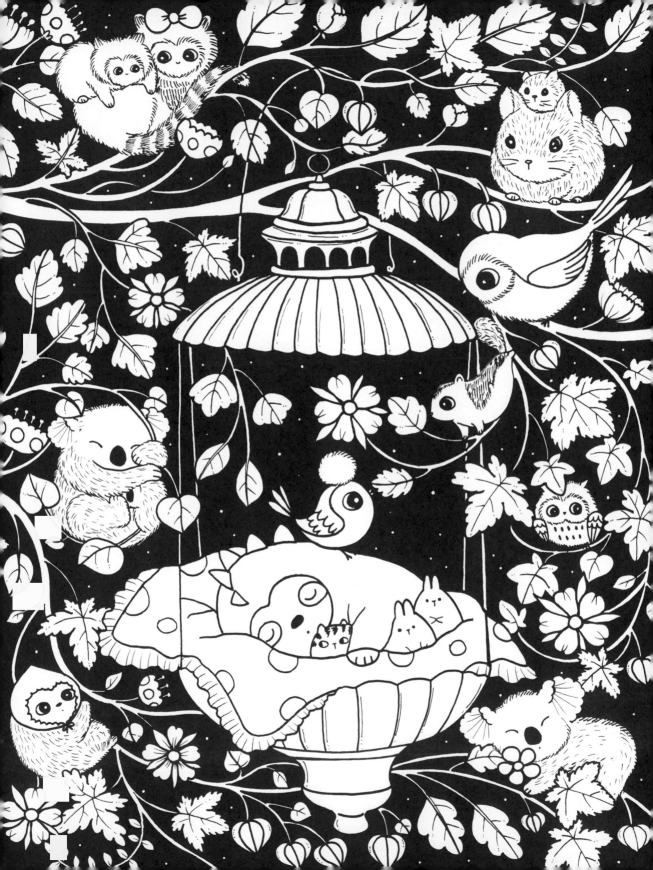

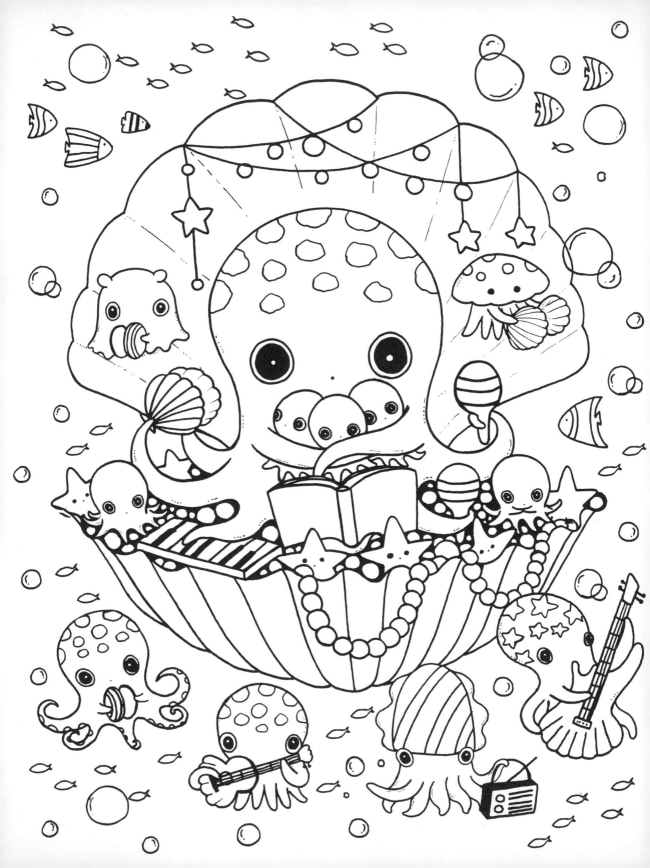

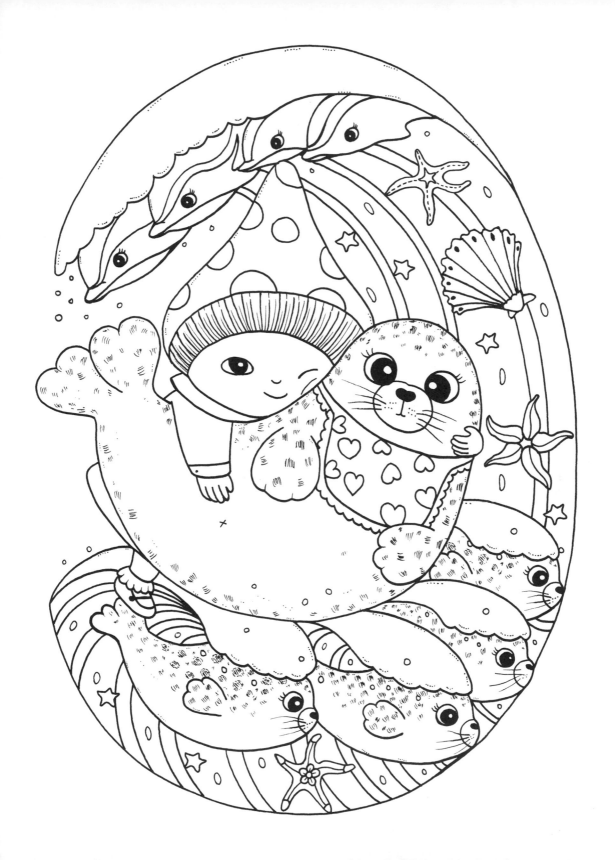

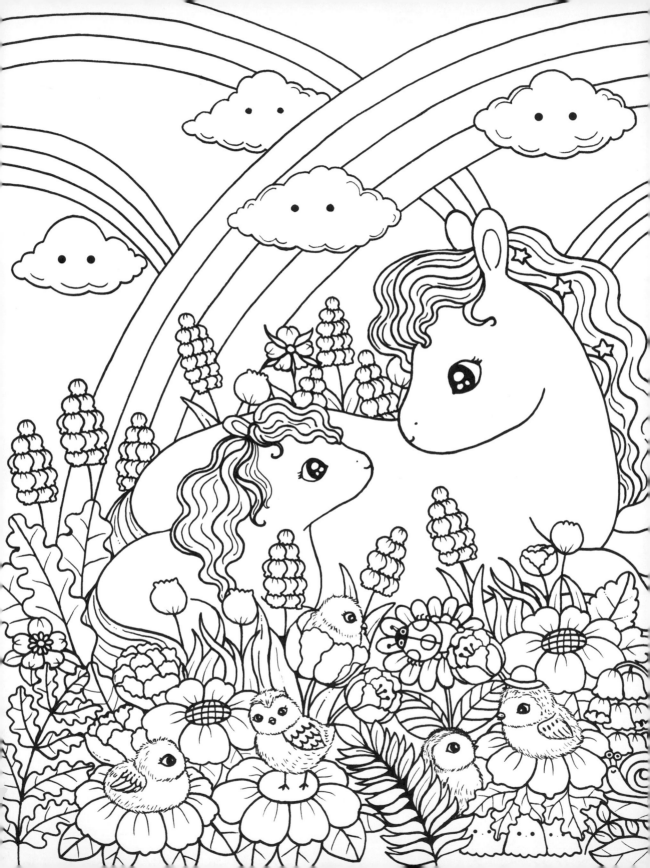

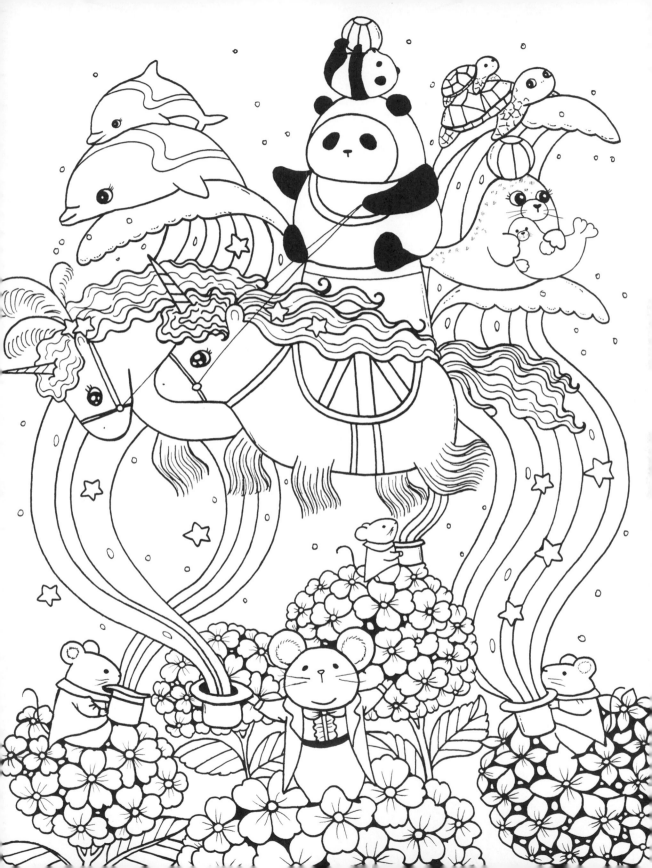

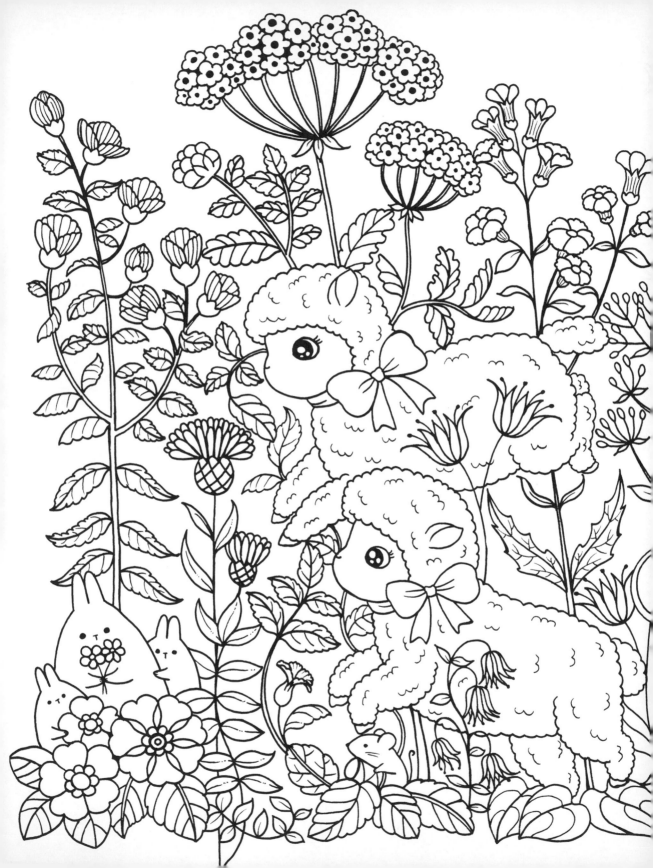

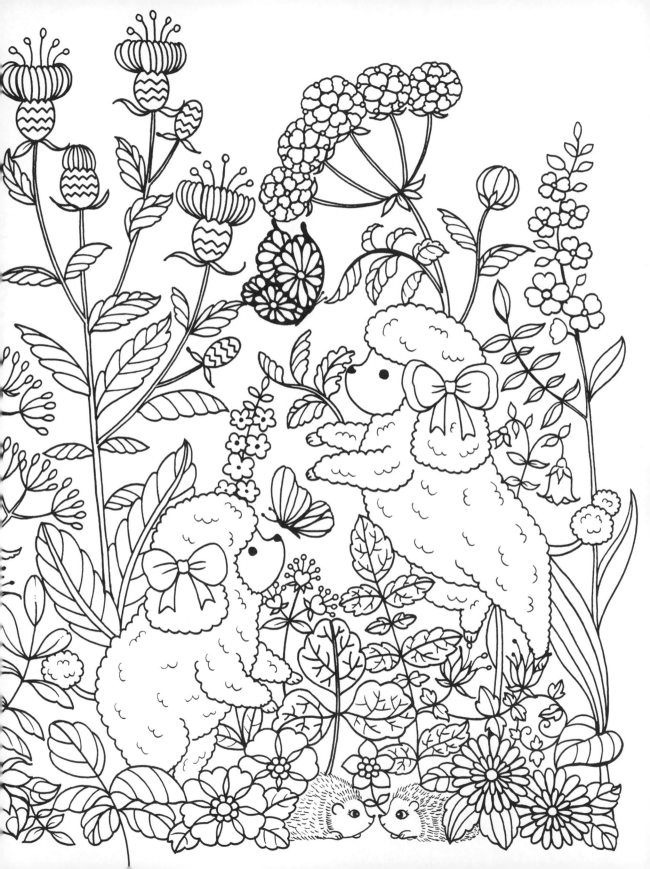

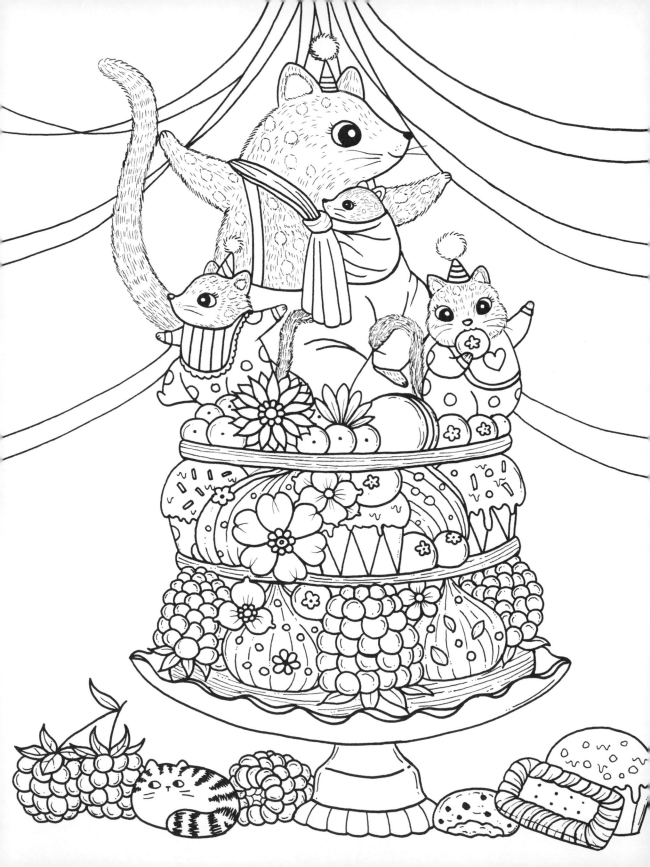

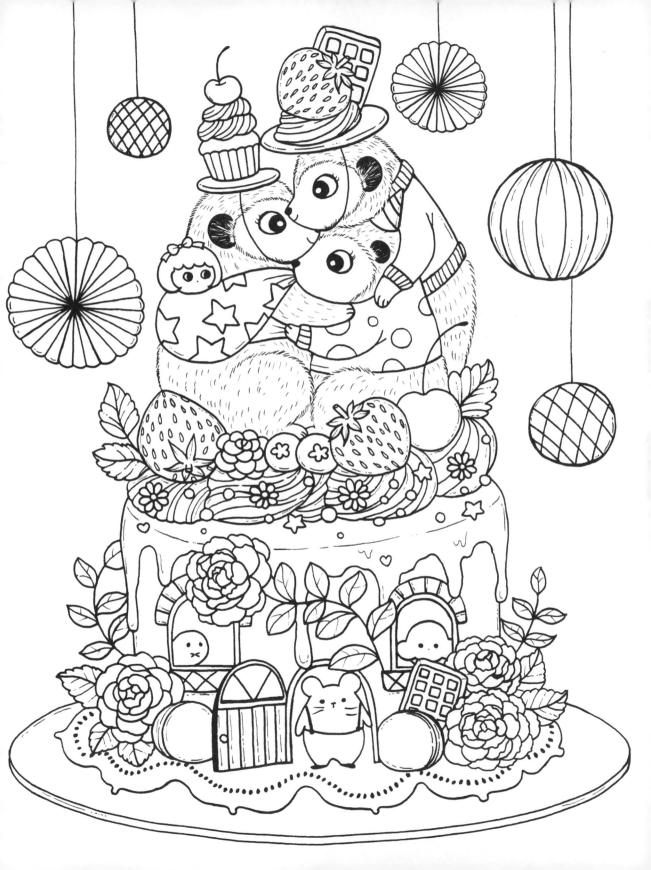

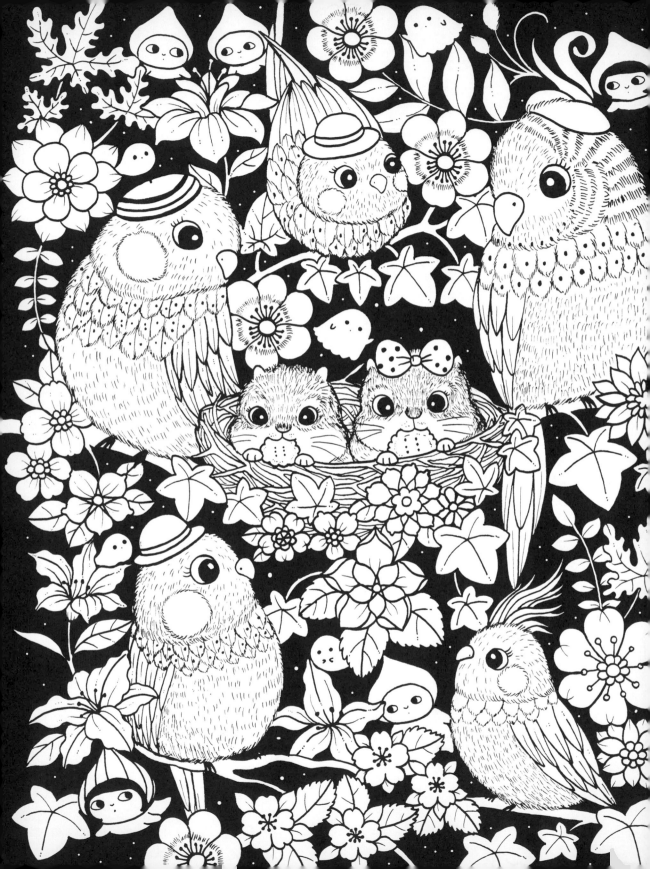

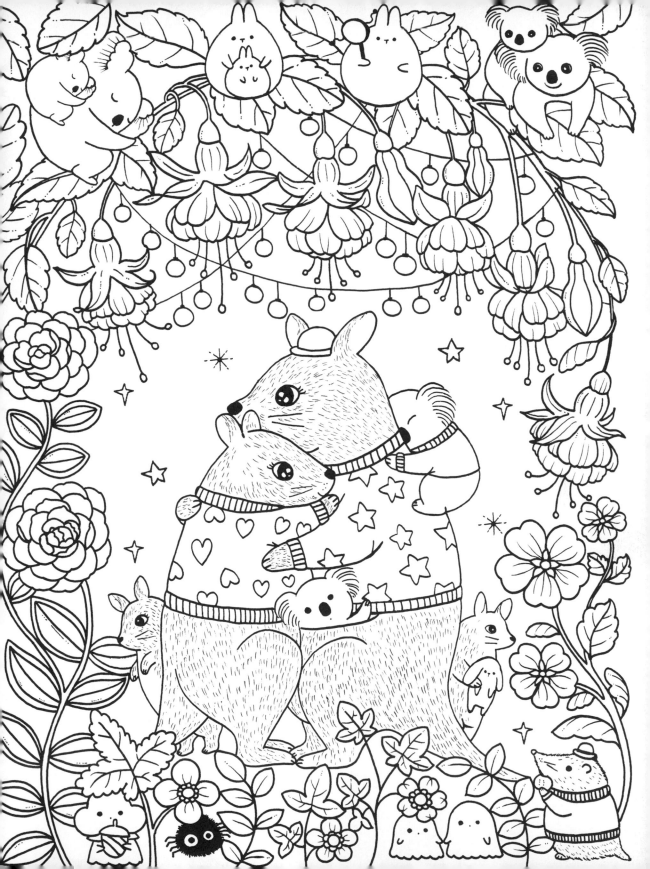

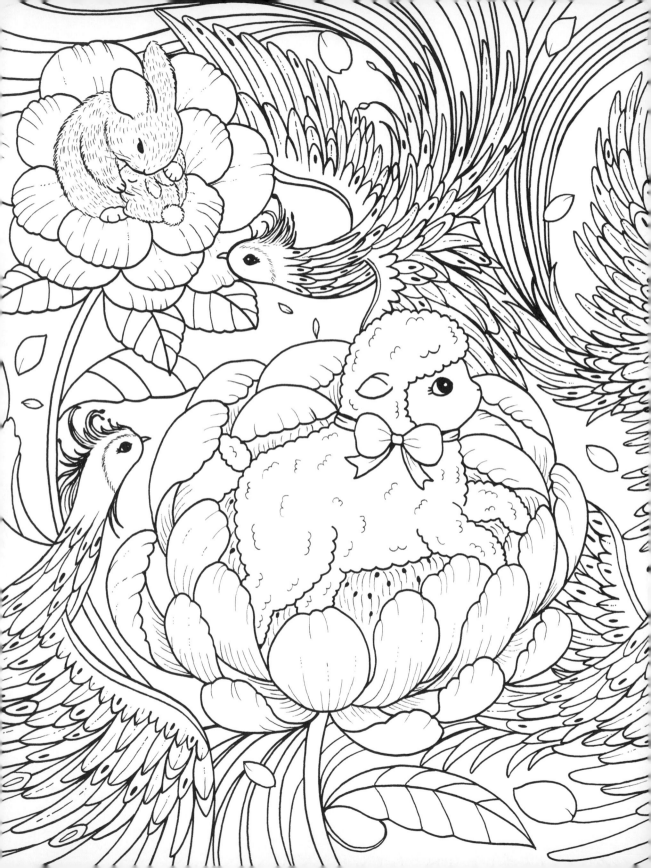

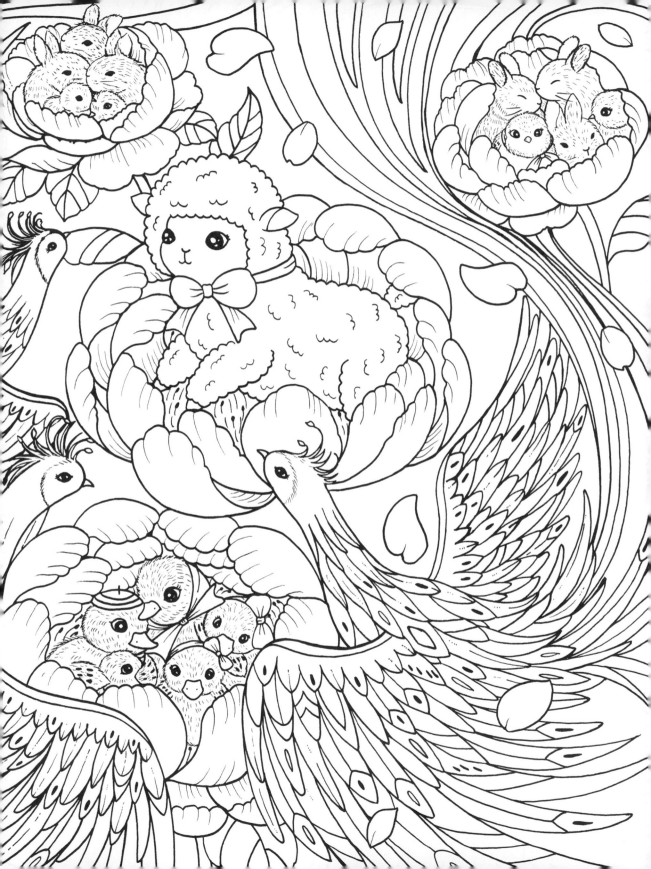

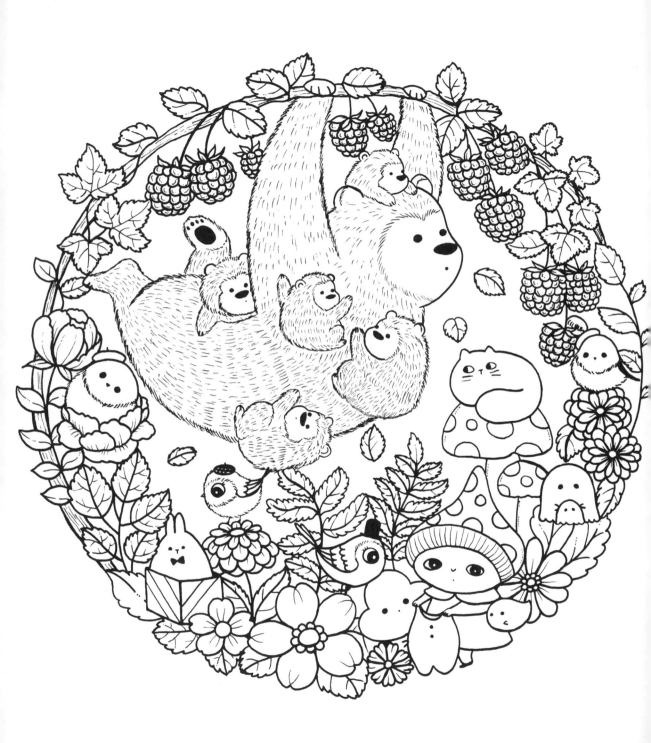

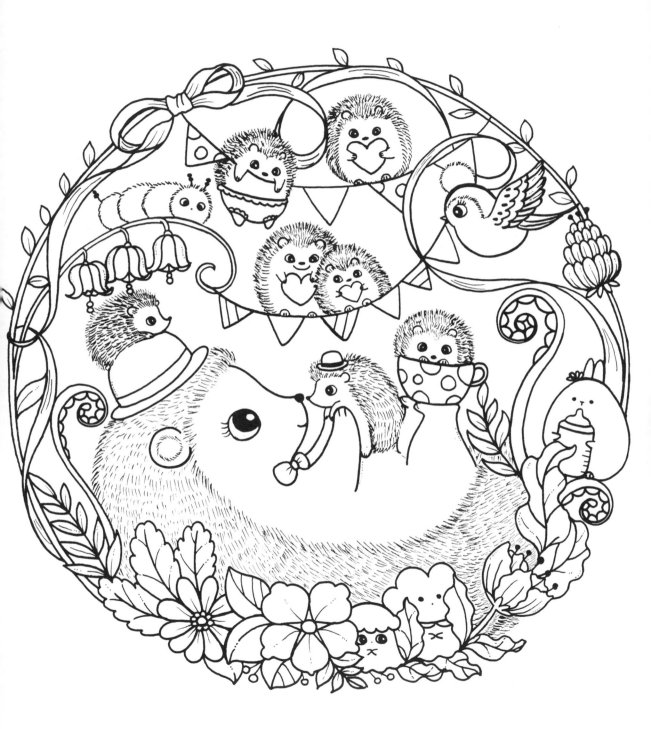

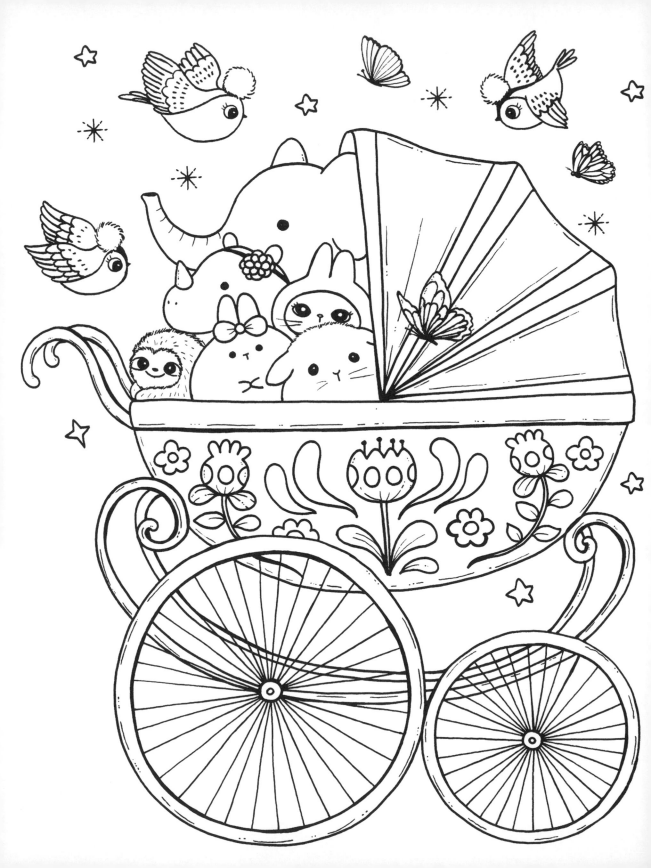

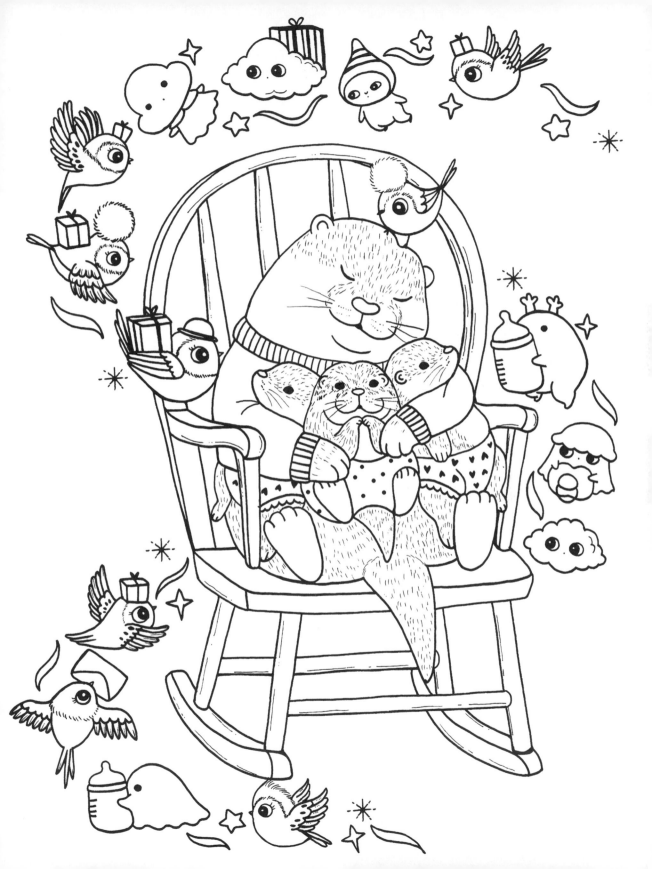

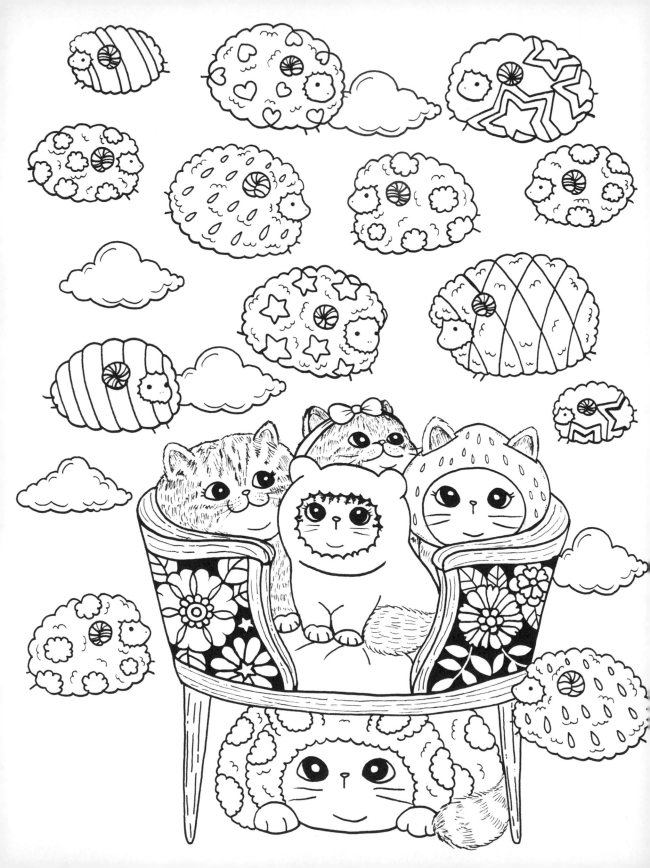

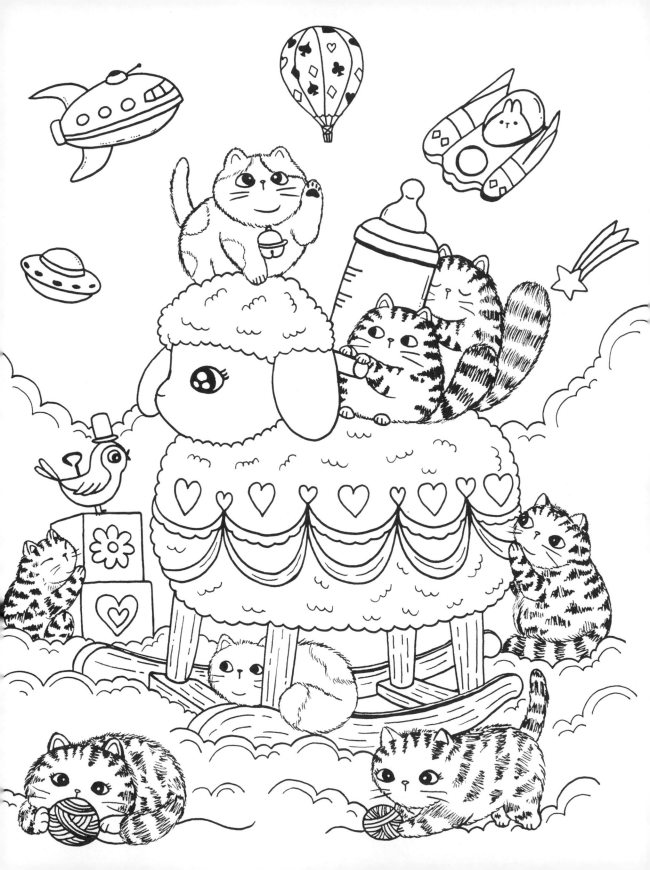

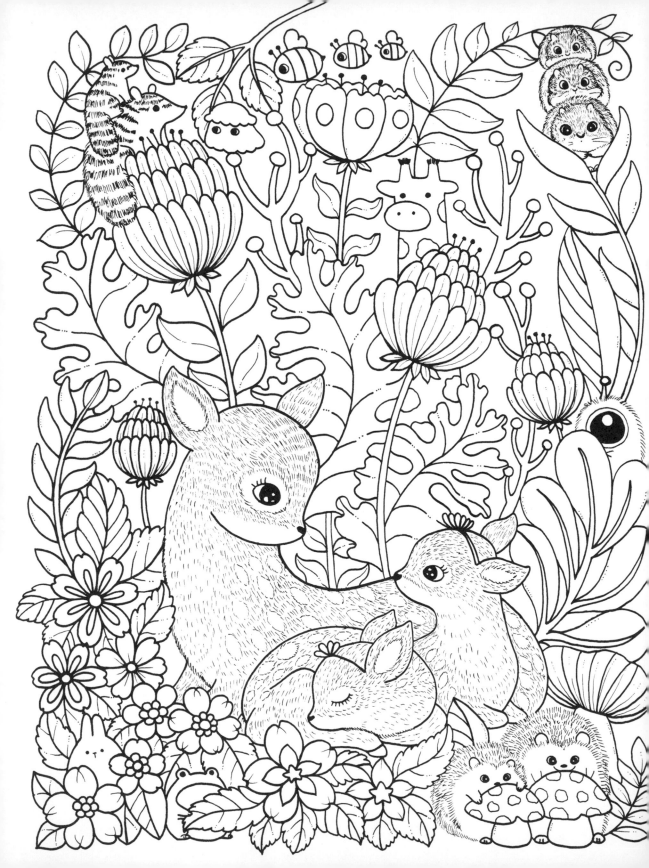

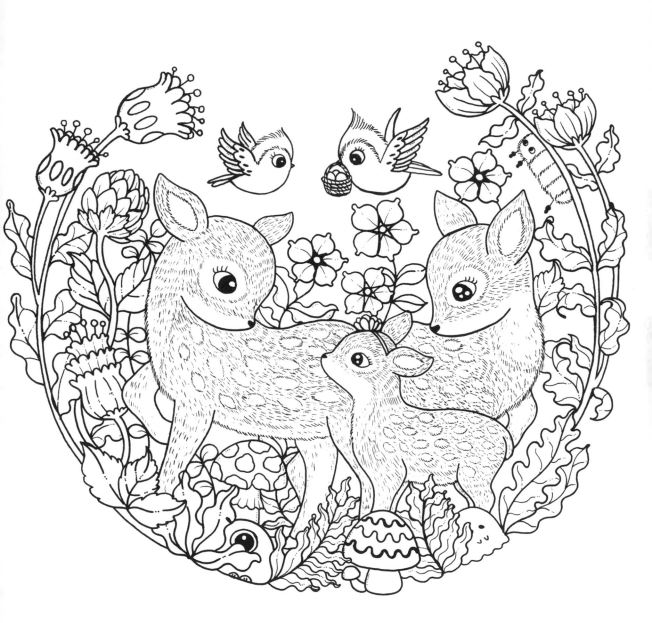

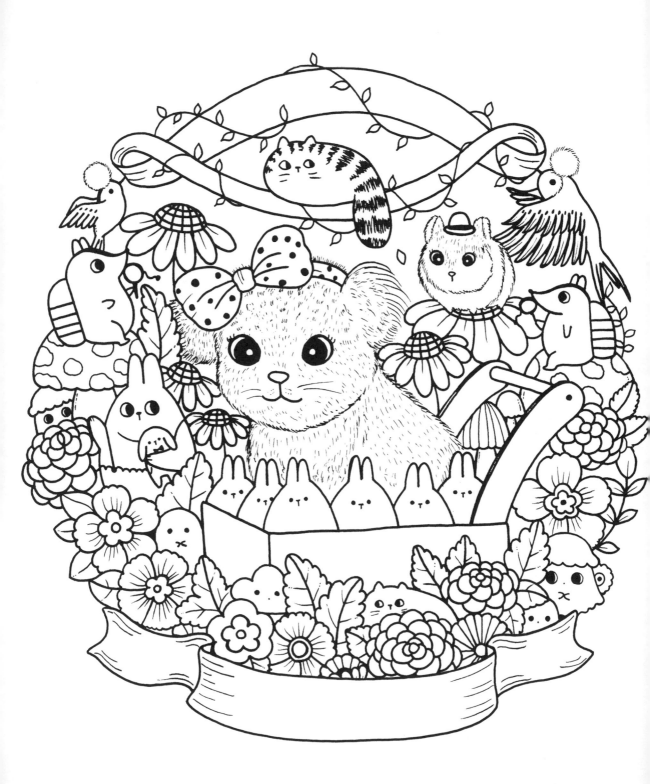

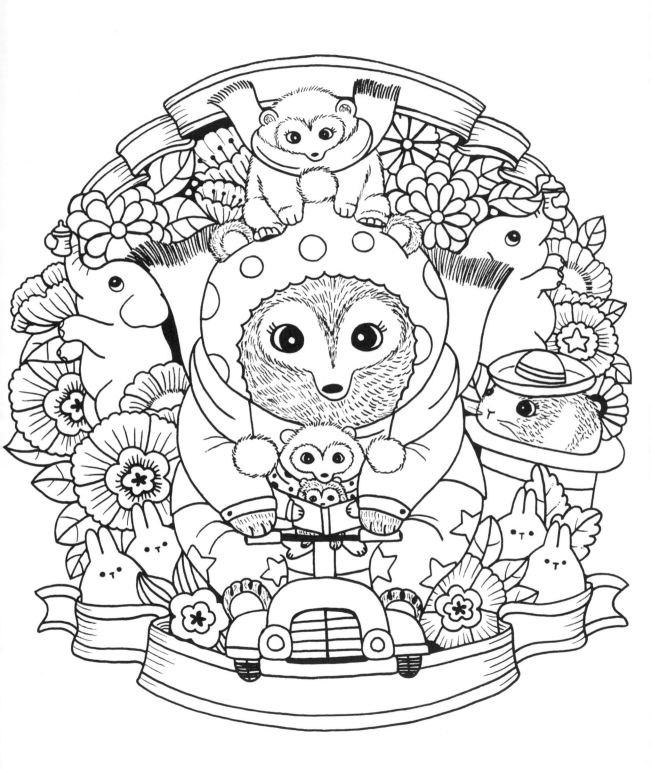

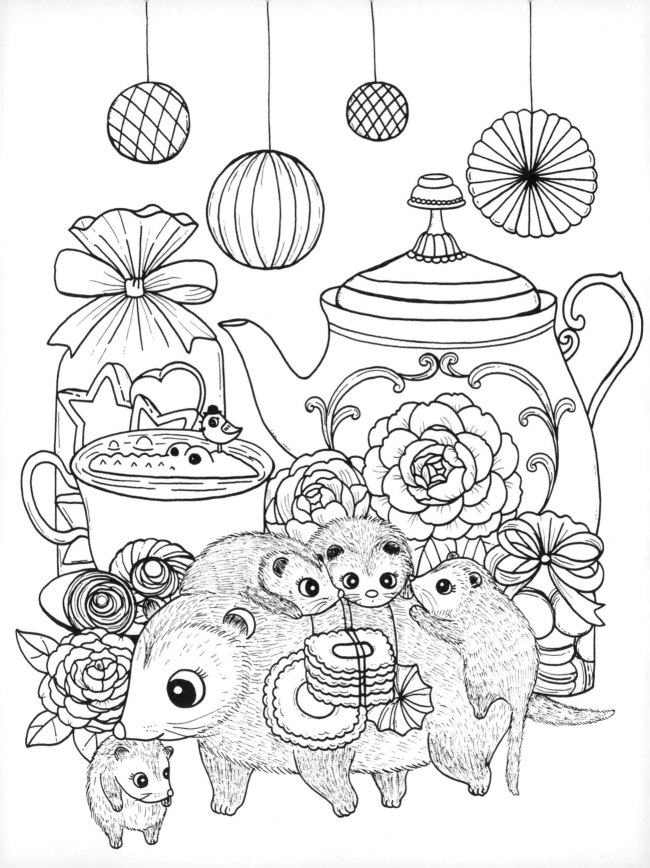

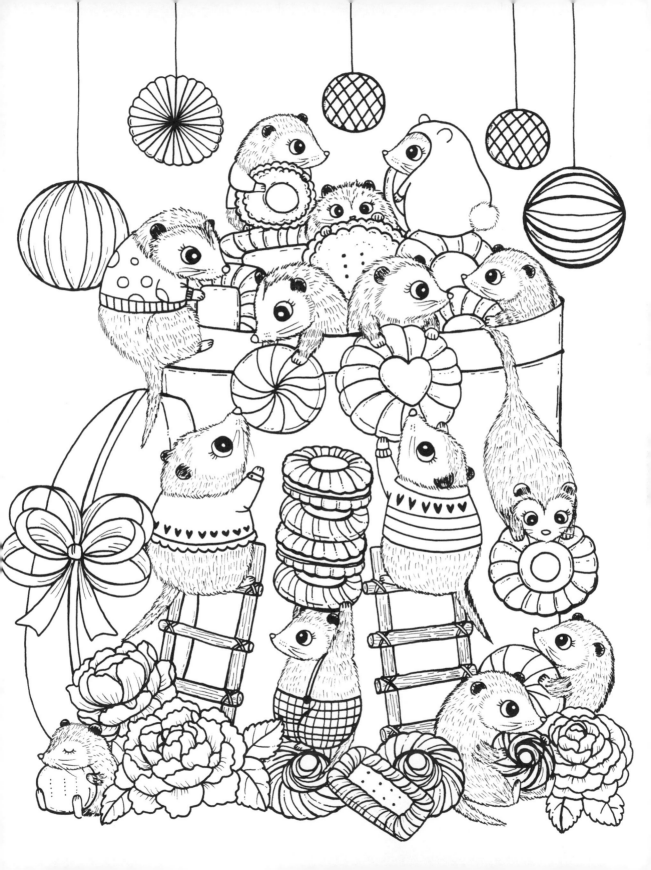

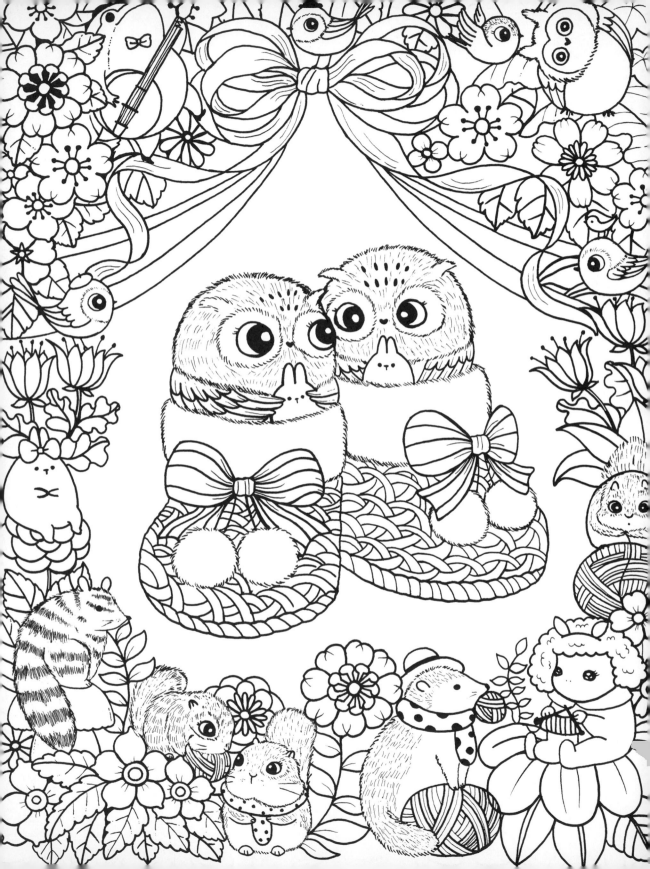

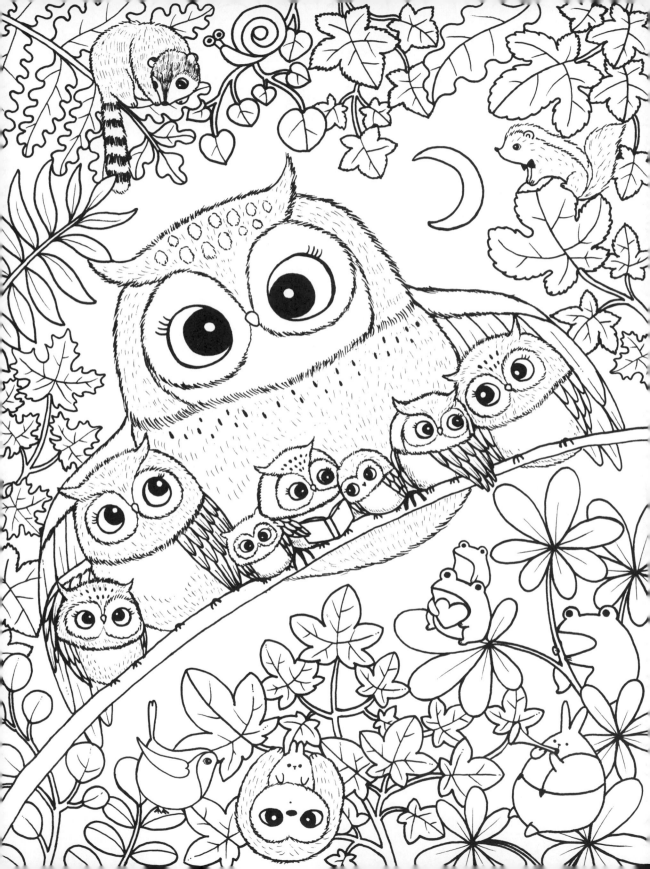

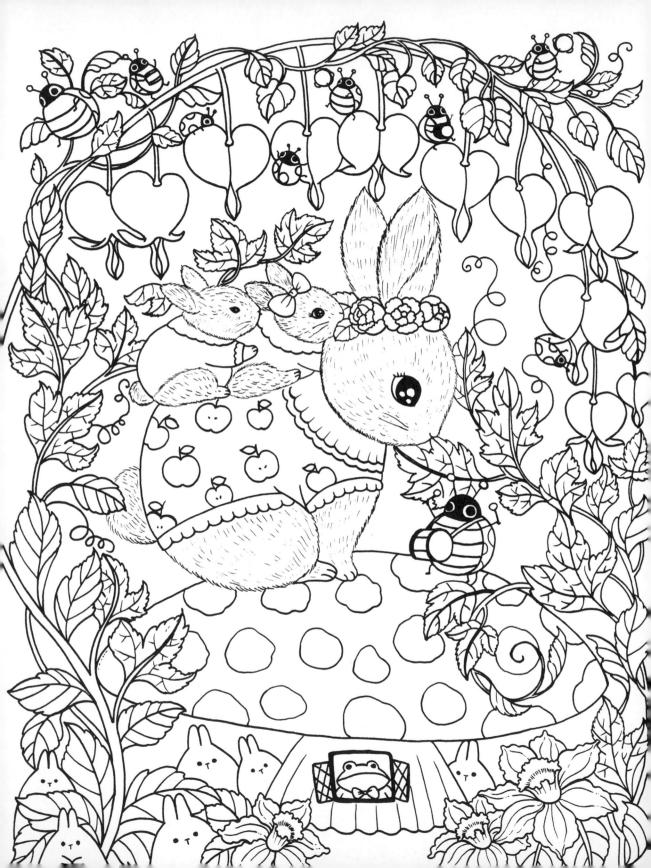

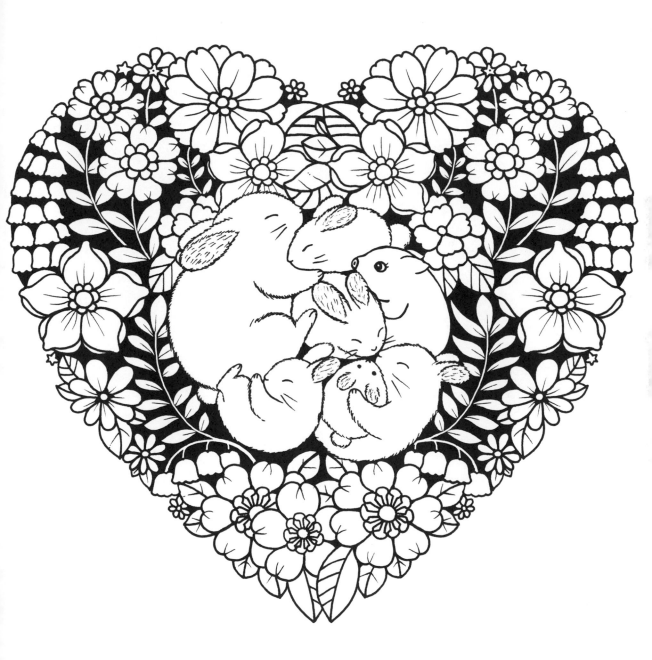

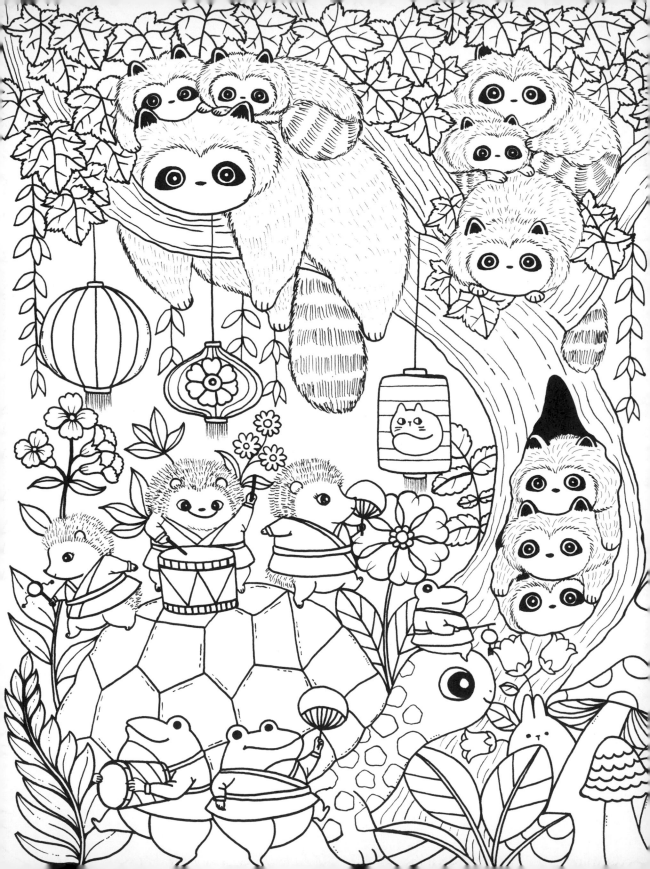

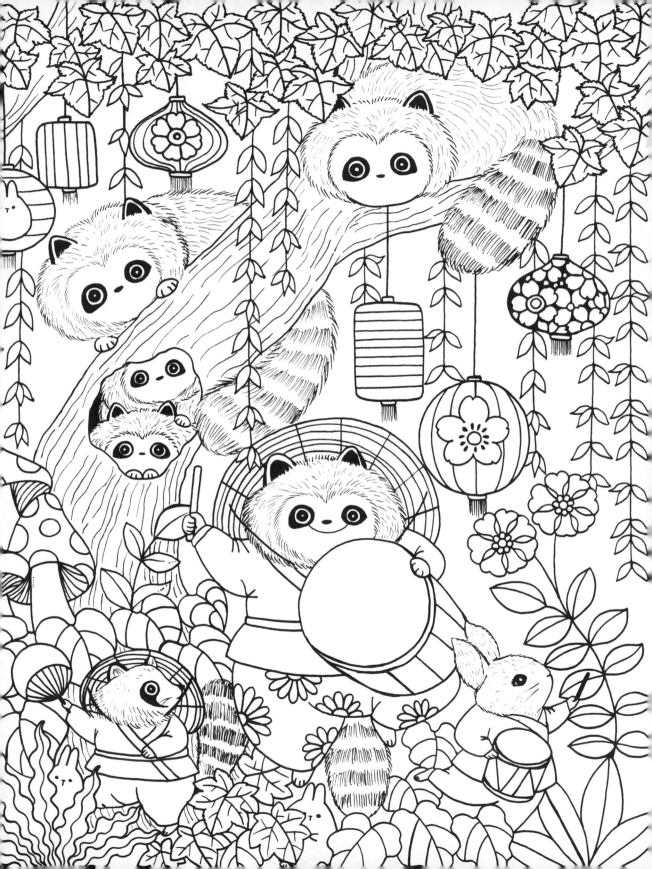

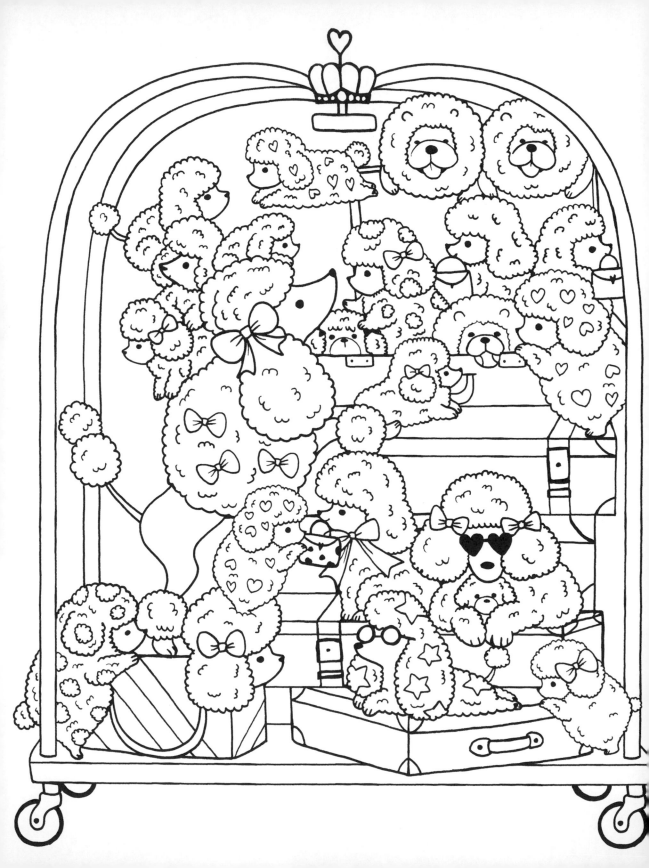

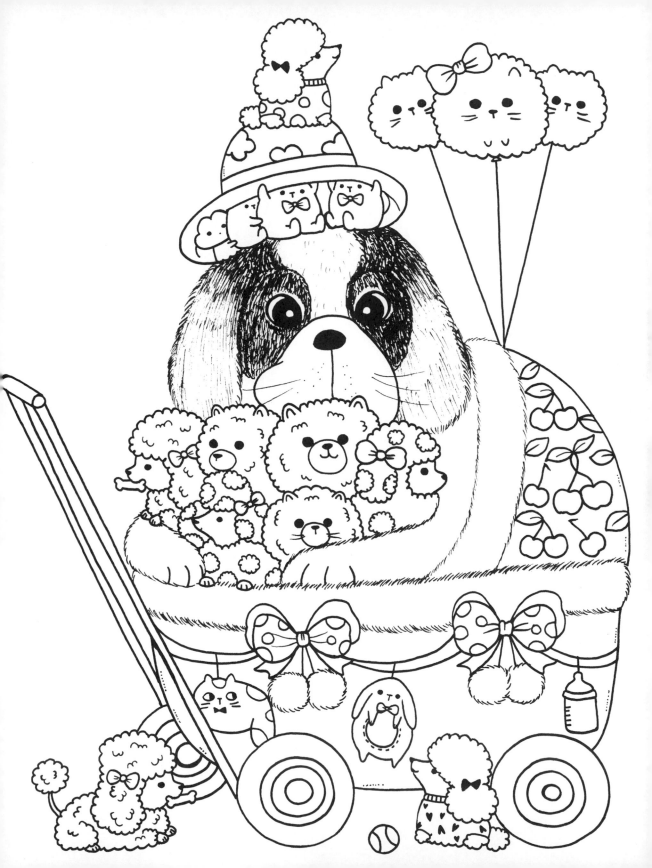

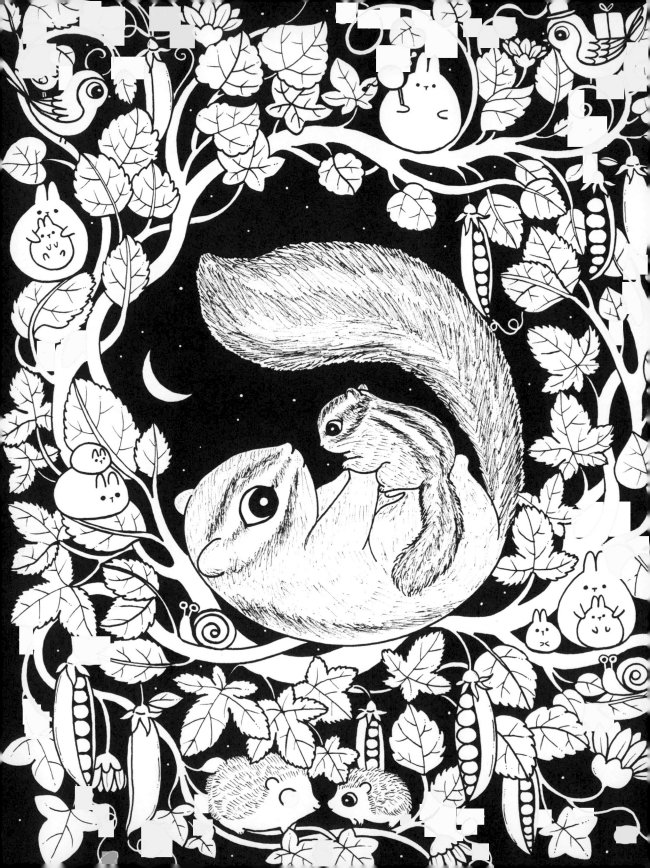

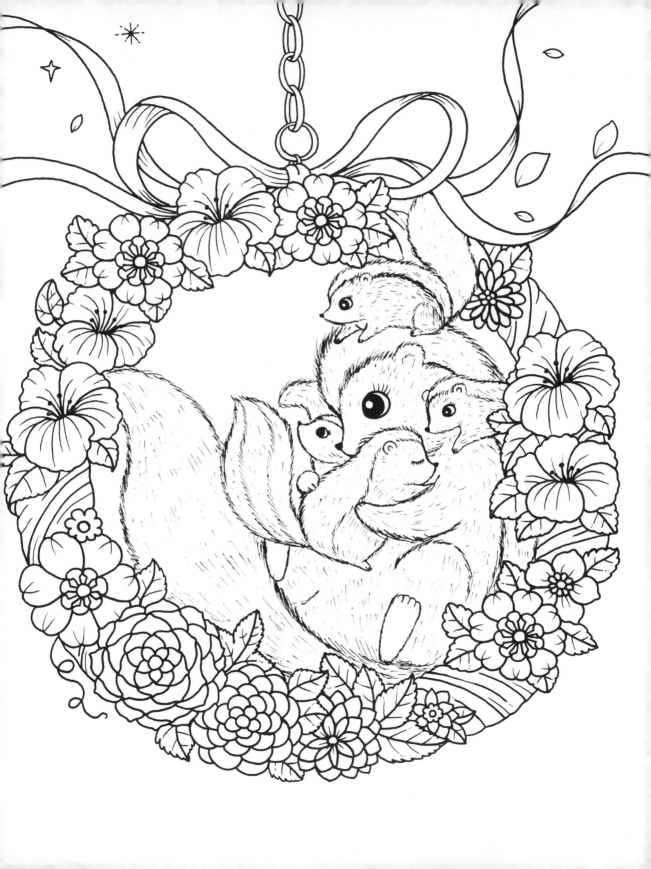

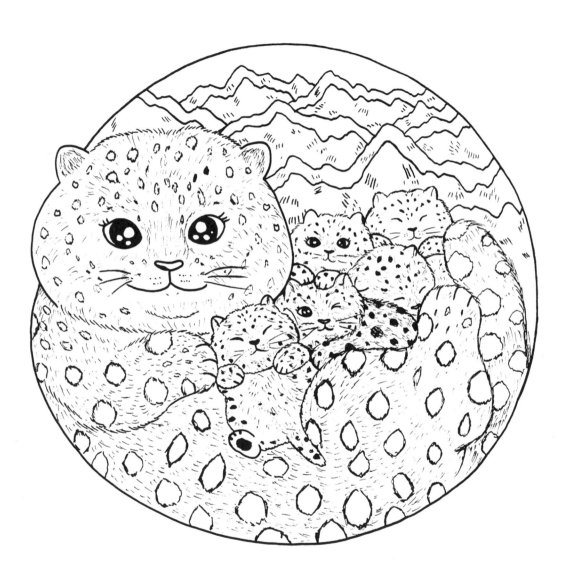